The Vitamin B12 Solution

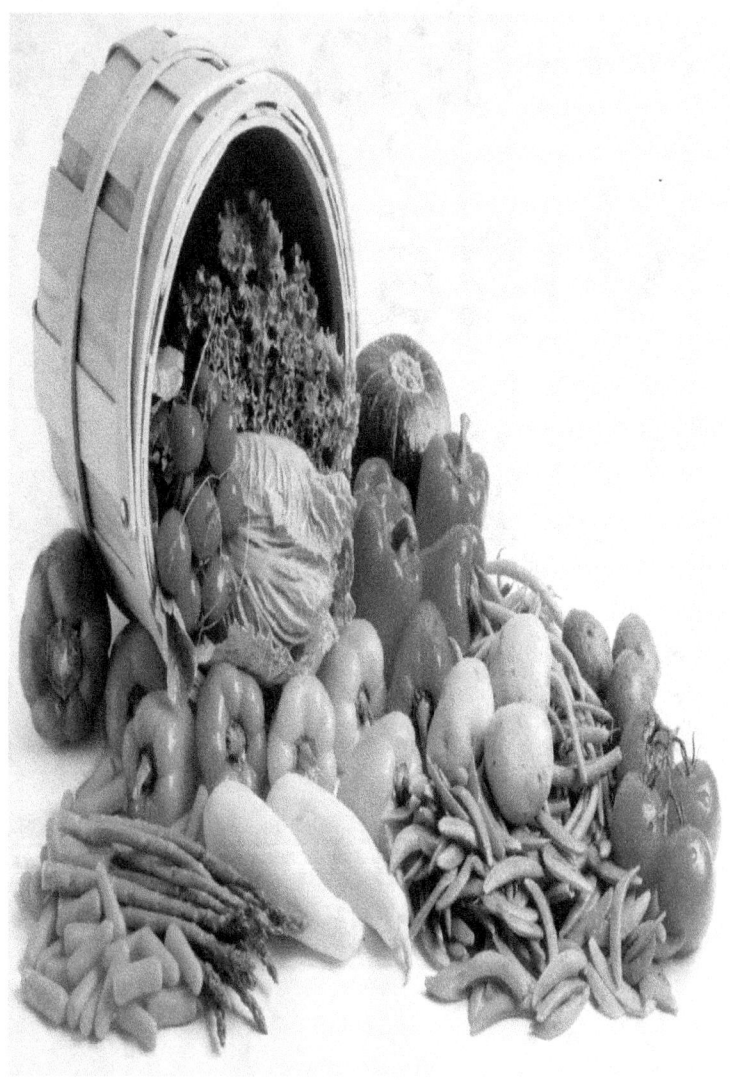

Rossie C Pattison

The Vitamin B12 Solution

Your Essential Key To Healthy Red Blood Cells And Anemia

Rossie C Pattison

Copyright Notice

Contents

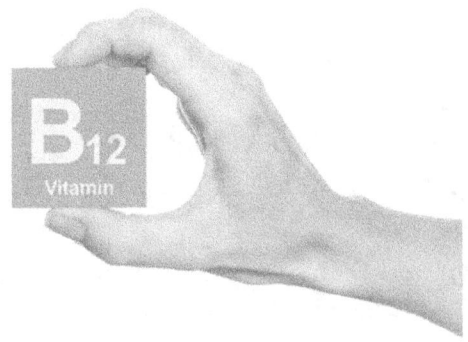

Preface: The Heart Pumping Station

The heart "pumping station" for the blood is the most dramatic organ in the body. It is the most talked-about, most written-about of all our vital organs. Poets, novelists and doctors have written millions of words about the "throbbing" heart, the "broken" heart, and the "diseased" heart. Everyone has a spleen and a liver as well as a heart, yet how many of us are made instantly conscious of these organs by the mere mention of them? Yet merely directing attention to the heart is enough to cause us to become immediately aware of its rhythmic beating and throbbing.

Since the heart, with all its functions and disorders, is "first page medical news," whatever is said or written about the human pump should be approached with caution and discretion. Usually the end product of most medical articles or books on the heart is not clarification, but more confusion in the mind of the victim of real or imaginary heart trouble. So-called "heart trouble" is not one simple disease, common to all heart sufferers. The heart is subject to as many distinct types of disorders and diseases as, for example, the lungs, or the eyes, or the sexual organs. Nor does the verdict "heart disease" necessarily mean an early death. Just as the diabetes patient must learn how to live with his disease, so the patient with the diseased heart must learn what will control and ease his ailment and then he must abide religiously by all the rules.

And the heart patient from whose turbulent mind stems the real cause for his disturbed heart action must learn to control his emotions! A little misinformation and a lot of imagination can produce a heart disorder as acute and as painful as that resulting from a genuinely diseased heart. Tom K. proved this to himself at the cost of much suffering and expense!

One day shortly after Tom's father had died of a heart attack; Tom felt a twinge of pain travel down his left arm. A knife-thrust could have caused him no greater horror. Heart trouble! It wasn't possible. Yet he was very much like his father in build and temperament, so probably he was also susceptible to the same illnesses.

Tom was only thirty two years old at the time, engaged to a lovely girl, and he certainly was not ready to die. Yet, if he were a "heart case," would it be fair to his intended wife to burden her with a husband apparently foredoomed either to early death or to years of semi-invalidism?

9

And his mother, still grieving for her husband what a cruel blow it would be to learn that her son must suffer the same fate. Deciding not to say anything for a while to his mother or to his sweetheart, Tom consulted a heart specialist and was referred to a public laboratory for an electro-cardiogram.

During the test the machine broke down twice and had to be jarred back into operation by the young lady (obviously quite new at her job) who was operating it. But she assured Tom that if the recording did not show up as having been correctly taken after being checked by the "head technician," she would re-do the test.

The recording, however, was passed as "all right," and the results were sent to Tom's physician. Yes, said the heart specialist after studying the electrocardiogram, it was evident that Tom had a heart disorder that needed careful watching. However, it did not appear to be a disturbance that would require bed rest unless the symptoms became more pronounced. He gave Tom a prescription for a mild heart stimulant, and dismissed him with a bit of good advice about "not worrying."

Tom tried not to worry. But what vigorous, robust young man would not be alarmed at suddenly finding himself the victim of an unsuspected heart ailment? So Tom worried. Within several weeks, he developed a pain in his chest so severe that every breath was an ordeal.

Blinding waves of dizziness and nausea made it impossible for him to continue working. No longer could he hide his condition from his mother or his sweetheart. The doctor was summoned posthaste. Six weeks' bed rest and a strong drug for the heart was his prescription. But at the end of six weeks, Tom's suffering as intense as ever, he remained flat on his back for another six weeks and still another.

By this time, Tom despaired of ever getting married, and he tried to break his engagement. But, fortunately for him, Tom's fiancée was a sensible girl. She agreed to release him, but only on condition he has another electro-cardiogram taken. Tom consented and went to the laboratory of a reputable hospital.

You've guessed it there was absolutely nothing wrong with Tom's heart but his imagination! The shock of his father's sudden death, combined with a wrong diagnosis based on the carelessly recorded first electrocardiogram, produced in Tom K. heart symptoms as real and as disabling as the symptoms suffered by a true victim of angina pectoris or coronary thrombosis.

Introduction

Heart Trouble – Jim's Story

Jim W. was a small man, wiry and active. But along about his forty-third year, he began puffing and panting at the slightest exertion. Even a short flight of stairs or a mild slope would leave Jim breathless. But he was not especially alarmed. He decided he was smoking too much and promised himself to "cut down" but, of course, went right on smoking as many cigarettes as ever. Then Jim developed an irritating, hacking cough. He told himself that now he surely would have to stop smoking. And he did for several months.

But the cough did not get any better, so Jim reasoned that since he already had contracted a "cigarette cough," evidently nothing could be done about it; he might as well enjoy himself, so he went out and bought a couple of packs of cigarettes. About now Jim developed other symptoms that took his mind on his breathlessness and his coughing. For no apparent reason, Jim would start vomiting. He also noticed a sore, extremely tender feeling, over his liver.

Before and after a meal he would feel "bloated." So Jim decided he was "bilious"! Patiently he submitted to the round of dosing that his wife put him through. But Jim's "biliousness" grew so much worse he had to remain away from his job. Then his ankles began swelling so he could not wear his shoes.

Off to the doctor went Jim at last, only to learn that his panting and his "biliousness," as well as his swollen ankles, were symptoms of a tired, inefficiently operating heart. The doctor called it "congestive heart failure."

He explained to Jim that, because of strain and fatigue, the heart muscle had so weakened that it could not completely empty all the blood at each pumping from the four heart chambers. Proper pressure cannot be maintained by a heart only half-emptied of its blood at each pumping; therefore, the blood being returned to the heart backs up in the veins, like water in a clogged drain, and seeps out into the nearby tissues.

Consequently, the blood seeping into the tissues caused his ankles to swell; the lung tissues became congested with blood, causing the shortness of breath and the persistent cough; the

13

tissues in the digestive system became so gorged with stagnant blood that they brought on vomiting and the congested area over the liver.

Jim's doctor also told him that, although congestive heart failure is a serious situation, it is not always a hopeless one. With an intelligent, co-operative understanding of his condition, any victim of this type of cardiac disorder can restore his heart to efficient operation.

But in between these two extremes of imaginary and real heart disease is a third type of heart victim the one whose overwrought, tense mind reacts directly on the heart, causing among other disorders the heart ailment known as angina pectoris literally, "pain of the chest."

The difference between the truly diseased heart and the emotionally harassed heart is that the first suffers actual physical degeneration, whereas the second is worried into a disorder by super-emotionalism.

Physicians whose patients come mainly from black or Chinese neighborhoods have noticed how seldom a victim of angina pectoris appears in their offices. The calm, placid temperament of these races does not promote this type of heart disease.

Primitive People

Among primitive people, too, the civilized curse of heart disease and high blood pressure is practically unknown.

Dr. Holden, famous American explorer-scientist, while cutting his way through miles of the Amazon jungle in Northern Brazil on a medical research mission, discovered that high blood pressure and all forms of heart disease are almost unknown among the natives.

These are Indians of the most primitive tribes who have had little or no contact with the white man and his civilization. They are a casual people who, like most aborigines, live from day to day, never driving themselves either physically or mentally.

During his travels in this thickest of all jungles, Dr. Holden examined hundreds of natives. He found absolutely no trace of heart trouble or hypertension (high blood pressure) in any of them, except for a few who were suffering from injuries.

Years ago the family doctor in a quiet community rarely was called upon to treat a case of angina pectoris. But today the heart specialist in a prosperous, metropolitan neighborhood inhabited by business and professional men and women can record his angina pectoris patients by the dozens.

Although angina pectoris is not the only heart symptom suffered by the worrier, it is by the far the most painful. But no less annoying are disorders such as extra heartbeats, disturbed rhythm, increased rate of beat, and acute dilation all of them heart disturbances that may be brought on by violent emotion.

Actually there is no telling what an outburst of strong emotion or continuous outbursts may do by way of harming an otherwise normal heart.

Chapter 1

The Disturbed Mind

The case of Bessie W. is a good example of what a disturbed mind can do to the heart. For several years this forty-five year old woman had suffered acute attacks of heart palpitation. Her heart would beat so wildly she had the feeling of suffocating, and the attack would last for hours. During extremely violent sieges, her pulse would cease momentarily and she would have to be revived with injections of a strong heart stimulant.

The professional diagnosis was that Bessie was "approaching her menopause" and such palpitations were not unusual at this time. Bessie resigned herself to her fate. But she finally came under the care of a physician who suspected the true cause of Bessie's heart disorder.

It was Bessie's mind, and not any physical degeneration, that was whipping up her heart into these spells of wild beating. Not long after she had married, many years before, Bessie had entered into an extra-marital affair with a man who subsequently moved away from town, leaving Bessie sincerely repentant of her infidelity and resolved henceforward to be faithful to her husband.

Then, after years of apparent forgetfulness, a man moved into Bessie's neighborhood that bore a strong resemblance to her former lover. The very presence of this man served as an acute reminder of the grave injustice she had done many years before to her devoted husband.

The bottled-up sense of shame in Bessie's mind became so intense that her heart ultimately was affected by the emotional storms which raged in her thoughts every time she saw the man who resembled her past lover. Therefore, it was deep-seated emotion, not disease that made Bessie's heart palpitate so violently.

Cardiac Disturbance

Soldier's heart is another type of cardiac disturbance that has its origin in the mind rather than in physical degeneration. More than anyone else, a soldier is subjected constantly to intense emotional upsets and adjustments homesickness, anger, fear, horror.

Such constant waves of intense emotions leave their mark on his heart by causing rapid heartbeat, pains in the heart region, abnormal sweating and flushing, breathlessness, or equally disturbing symptoms. However, for the most part, when the soldier is demobilized or relieved of active duty, these heart disturbances clear up immediately.

The Best Treatment

The best treatment for the victim of a mind-induced heart ailment is to make him or her realize that the trouble is not caused by any breakdown in the cardiac organ itself; rather he should be impressed with the fact that the disturbance can be traced directly to an intense mental condition.

And once the patient can be made to realize the truth, his heart disorder will improve greatly provided, of course, he also strengthens his brain cells to the point where they do not again allow morbid thinking to gain the upper hand in his mind.

If you are a "heart patient," do any of these emotions fit your case?

A famous heart specialist has listed these as some of the intense emotional conditions which are most likely to cause the heart to go on a rampage:

- An overwhelming frustration brought on by the sense of unending obligation an endless procession of things that must be done.

- A bitter conflict between duty and desire a burning desire to do one thing, only to be held back by a strong sense of duty.

- A hopeless sense of defeatism a feeling of "it can't be done, what's the use."

- A feeling of impotence when confronted by an apparently "unsolvable" problem a sensation of "beating against the bars" with no hope of getting anywhere.

- An attitude of self-pity a feeling that "nobody loves me, everybody picks on me."

- A habit of living in the past a tendency to dwell on what "might have been."

- A sense of futility a feeling of being no longer needed, of being "put on the shelf."

- An inner rebellion at being dominated an unfulfilled desire to tell someone of!

- A sensation of fear an unreasoning harboring of anxiety, dread or terror lest something happen or not happen.

Chapter 2

Diet and Supplements

Diet and certain supplements have proved worthwhile in the prevention and treatment of heart disorders. I shall describe these in detail a little later. But first there are definite, inevitable mental attitudes which the heart patient true, false or potential must resolve to adopt before any type of therapy can do him much good. The heart patient's philosophy can be boiled down to this:

"Tomorrow is another day; there's nothing I must do now. For what will it matter a hundred years from now? I'll let the other fellow do the worrying!" The worrier must learn that nothing in this world is ever perfect, and that no person ever lived who was completely without some troubles and vexations.

It has been said that if everyone in the world could throw his troubles onto a pile and choose another set from those already discarded by someone else, most of us would walk away again with our own troubles!

There is great wisdom in this as well as potent healing properties for the victims of mind-induced heart disturbances. None of us is as important or as perfect as we like to imagine; nor is anything as terrible as we picture it.

Very seldom is a personal problem so serious that it cannot be lightened by a sense of humor, and a willingness to co-operate with others! The person who can laugh at himself is not likely to end up in the office of the heart specialist or the psychiatrist.

Perhaps a quick look at the heart itself will help dispel the awesome mystery that surrounds this hard-working organ. The heart is one of the most efficient machines ever devised. Every day it beats approximately 100,000 times.

During every year it makes over 37 million contractions. In a person seventy years of age, this means that the heart has contracted over three billion times and has pumped something like 40 million gallons of blood that carries oxygen and nourishment to the body cells and removes poisonous wastes from them, as well as answering emergency calls for rush blood to any organ or muscle.

When one stops to consider that the modern, highly efficient auto-mobile motor will rarely go more than 50,000 miles without repairs or replacements of some sort, we marvel all the more at the efficiency of the cardiac "motor" when we realize that in the average person the heart functions without repairs or replacements for the equivalent of a million miles of driving!

The comparison is all the more astounding when we take this into consideration: The motor in our car does not run continually, yet our hearts must work on and on, apparently without resting.

The heart does manage to snatch a split second of rest between beats but only when the average is 72 beats a minute. A heartbeat above this rate does not give the heart a chance to pause to "catch its breath." Therefore a rapidly beating heart is a laboring heart, like a runner dashing pell-mell uphill with never a pause for breath.

Nor would we wish to take away from the heart this ability to speed up. For it is this ability that allows us to exercise, or to protect ourselves in times of danger when rapid, agile movements are imperative, or when quick thinking is needed.

The heart is so constructed that it can provide "extra current" whenever the load is heavy, the same as the electric company's power plants are equipped to supply extra power instantly to meet unusual consumer demands such as arise from a suddenly darkened sky.

The greater amount of blood sent coursing through the blood vessels is needed to supply the tissues with "energy" in the form of the greater amount of oxygen brought to them by the more rapidly traveling red blood cells.

Unlike the electrical power station, however, that can throw the switches and cut in more dynamos, the heart must meet its increased demands with the same machinery the red blood cells and it does this by speeding up their rate of travel throughout the arteries and veins.

Therefore, it is easy to understand why, after the heart has answered the cry of "Wolf, wolf!" minute after minute, hour after hour, day after day, it becomes weary.

Yet this faithful organ never refuses to keep sending out blood in rush quantities, until that fatal moment when it no longer is physically capable of keeping up the pace.

Unfortunately, the heart has no way of knowing whether the distress signals it gets from the brain are the "real McCoy" or whether they are frauds.

The heart works just as speedily to answer the cry of danger when we must act in a bonafide emergency, as it does when we merely imagine ourselves in some peril. That is why continual emotional upsets place so severe a strain on the heart; the cry "Help, help!" keeps coming from the mind, and the heart keeps responding.

Excitement, anger, fear, hatred, frustration all these place as great a strain on the heart as strenuous physical exercise. In other words, you may sit quietly in an armchair, and yet overwork your heart by "racing" your emotions. Shaped something like a pear, with the point or apex lying low in the chest about three inches to the left of the middle line of the chest, the heart has for its neighbors the lungs and the stomach.

The lower tip, or point, of the heart touches the wall of the chest between the fifth and sixth ribs on the left side, and slightly inside the nipple of the left breast. The broader, upper part of the heart lies high up in the chest behind the breastbone, level with the space between the second and third ribs. Here also are suspended certain other large blood vessels such as the aorta, the main artery.

The heart itself is a hollow muscle. We are accustomed to thinking of the arm or leg muscles, but seldom does anyone stop to consider that the heart is made of approximately the same muscle fibers as those that comprise the lifting and flexing mechanism in the arms, hands or legs.

On second thought, it does not seem so strange that the heart should be nothing more nor less than a muscle, for its entire function is purely muscular. It contracts, squeezing the blood from the four heart chambers into the arteries, and then it relaxes, allowing the "oxygen-recharged" blood to flow into the chambers preparatory to the next dispatch of blood throughout the arteries.

26

And so on, contracting and relaxing, with only that split second of rest in between provided we do not force it to beat over 72 times a minute. Remember, then, that the heart is a muscle. And all the while it is pumping blood throughout the body to feed and cleanse other muscle cells, it must maintain an adequate supply of blood to nourish and purify its own muscle.

This is done by means of the coronary arteries. But when the heart muscle fails to get enough blood, it becomes cramped and diseased, just as any other muscle throughout the body. To simplify the comparison of the heart as a muscle with the muscles of the arm or leg, I spoke of its contracting and relaxing, something like the opening and shutting of a clenched fist. Actually, however, the action of the heart muscle is a little more complicated.

Each heartbeat occurs as a wave of contractions, beginning at the mouths of the great incoming veins, passing through the upper heart chambers (auricles), into the lower chambers (ventricles), and ending at the lower point of the heart (apex). Perhaps the comparison of this movement with the series of ripples started on the surface of a pond by a pebble would more nearly approximate this wave of contractions that constitute the heartbeat.

The rate of heartbeat is largely regulated by the carbonic acid content of the blood. Carbonic acid is the by-product of muscular action;

carbonic acid is the goad that speeds the heart into greater effort.

Chapter 3

Carbonic Acid Content in the Blood

A man digging ditches all day will have high carbonic acid content in his blood, produced by his muscles, in order to keep the heart supplying them with the necessary blood. However, when the ditch digger reaches home and sits quietly before the radio reading his paper, the carbonic acid content of his blood decreases greatly and his heart is allowed to slow down, thereby obtaining those split seconds of rest between beats.

From this anyone can readily understand why, when a heart patient is told to rest, it means complete immobility of the body. The entire purpose of the rest treatment is to inactivate the muscles of the body so completely that they cannot produce enough carbonic acid to speed up an already tired, overworked heart.

To give you some idea of the extra demands put upon the heart by exercise, when an emotionally calm person is resting in a prone position the heart pumps about three and a half quarts of blood through the arteries each minute.

But when that same person exercises hurries up and down stairs, for instance the spurt of carbonic acid produced by the muscles forces the heart to pump about five and a half quarts of blood per minute, or 60 percent more than while the body is lying at rest. Now, if that person is also laboring under some emotional strain while exercising, his heart must pump 70 percent more blood than while he is at rest.

This can be explained by the fact that, in addition to the blood needed for the actual physical exertion, there is an extra amount sent out by the heart to answer that false cry of "Help, help!" which the emotions keep broadcasting.

That is why heart failure so often results from strenuous exercise or extreme fatigue at a time when the victim is also laboring under a great emotional strain. I am thinking of the mother whose only daughter was being married to a man whom the mother violently disliked. However, she determined to say nothing, and set about giving the girl a beautiful home wedding.

For days the mother cleaned and scrubbed and sewed and baked, only to collapse from a fatal heart attack as she was dressing for the ceremony. The strain of the mother's grief, added to the extra physical exertion, was just too much for her heart.

But carbonic acid is not the only thing that accelerates the heart. The nerves which connect the heart directly with the central nervous system in the brain can also act as a spur to goad the heart into faster action, as in the case of the unfortunate mother who died at her daughter's wedding.

This nerve acceleration can cause a type of cardiac disorder known as "nervous heart." Organically the heart may be one hundred percent healthy, but it reacts abnormally to the stimulation of these heart nerves. Physicians recognize that a person with a nervous heart may suffer as much as, sometimes more than a person who suffers from some serious degeneration of the heart muscle.

While the heart itself is not sick, it is "nervous"; it resembles an automobile in good running condition, but managed by an excitable driver. Of course, in such cases, the victims are not afflicted with genuine disease; their trouble, as we have seen earlier, is purely of the mind.

Such persons are often aware of a deep sense of frustration, envy, dissatisfaction, hatred or fear, yet seldom do they realize what these strong, unbridled emotions are doing to their hearts. If the heart could be said to contain a "bottleneck," it would be in the coronary arteries

31

that supply the heart muscle itself with oxygen via the red blood cells.

When the blood channels in the heart muscle grow thick and narrow because the arterial walls are hardening, the heart muscles receive less and less nourishment. The old law of supply and demand affects the heart muscle the same as anything else. When less and less food is made available to a group of people, their ability to perform strenuous work decreases then disappears entirely.

And so it is with the heart. The pain of true angina pectoris is a warning that the heart muscle is not receiving enough blood nourishment to enable it to stand up under the usual exertions of its allotted task. In other words, the heart muscle suffers a cramp.

Chapter 4

Heart Ailments

Heart ailments are generally thought of as belonging to the middle years or to old age. This is true mostly of organic heart disease, that is, disease caused by actual physical degeneration of the cardiac muscle. But functional heart disturbances, that is, disorders of purely mental or nervous origin, are likely to strike at any time, particularly the eighteen to thirty five year old group.

Why? Because at this time of life, emotions generally are at fever pitch, and everything that happens to us during these years seems a hundredfold more important than it will later on in life's journey. Especially are young pregnant women, or young mothers, susceptible to functional heart ailments. Should these women develop what they believe to be a serious heart condition, they should waste no time in determining whether the disorder is functional or organic that is, false or true.

Without any thought of disparaging the skill of the hundreds of reputable physicians qualified to detect true or false heart disease, I would like to caution against accepting without reservation the first diagnosis. If possible, get the opinion of at least three competent physicians.

Vitamin E

No chapter on diseases of the heart would be complete without reporting the outstanding work being done by three Canadian doctors in treating heart diseases with vitamin E. Although some of the medical profession has looked askance at this method of treatment, the Drs. Evan and Wilfred Shute and Dr. Vogel sang have obtained astonishing results with dozens of patients who received extraordinary relief after being given heavy doses of a highly concentrated vitamin E.

Hundreds of the more than 4,000 patients whom these doctors have treated so far with vitamin E have been restored to health. Serious symptoms such as swollen feet and legs, breathlessness at the slightest exertion, and stabbing pains in the chest have disappeared after the treatment.

One patient, who formerly became breathless merely from walking across the room, can now get out the lawn mower and cut the grass. Another patient who could not walk a block without suffering agonizing pains in the chest can now play golf. After treating a patient with vitamin E, these three doctors claim they have heard, through the stethoscope, the sounds made by sick hearts turn into the healthy rhythm of a normal heart.

How did these doctors discover vitamin E as a heart remedy? A medical student, investigating the action of vitamin E in counteracting the hemorrhaging effects of estrogen, reported to Dr. Shute that dogs given injections of estrogen developed purple patches under the skin.

These were caused by a breaking down of the blood vessels. But after the dogs were given liberal doses of vitamin E, the purple patches cleared up.

Dr. Shute passed this knowledge along to Dr. Vogelsang who had as a patient a sixty-seven-year-old man suffering from hypertensive (caused by high blood pressure) heart disease, who was scheduled to undergo an operation for another ailment.

However, the patient's condition was so poor that Dr. Vogelsang was afraid to operate. The man's kidneys were barely functioning, his legs were badly swollen and ruptured blood vessels under the skin had covered his body with large purple patches.

Since vitamin E had cleared up the purple patches in the laboratory animals, why not try it on this patient? Each day the old man was given large doses of highly concentrated vitamin E.

On the fifth day after the treatment was started, Dr. Vogel sang visited his patient in the hospital only to find the bed empty. The old man was found helping the nurses carry trays! When reprimanded for getting out of bed, the old fellow replied that he hadn't felt so well in years. He was no longer breathless, and all swelling had disappeared from his feet and legs.

Proudly he boasted of having done more work that morning than he had for the past several years put together. From this experiment, Dr. Shute and Dr. Vogel sang concluded that vitamin E must exert some amazingly beneficial effect on the heart, as well as on the blood vessels themselves.

It was known at this time that vitamin E was a powerful stimulant to tired or diseased muscles. And what harder-working muscle is there in the entire body than the heart? That was it. Vitamin E was a perfect heart stimulant because it fed the muscle tissues. Previous research had shown that muscles starved of vitamin E needed several times the amount of oxygen required by healthy muscles.

Oxygen

This greater need for oxygen alone would whip up a diseased heart to the danger point. Therefore, if merely supplying all the vitamin E that the body muscles needed would cut down their oxygen requirements, the heart in addition to being properly nourished itself could slow down and take things easy.

The doctors were elated at the results obtained with this first patient yet almost afraid to hope for too great results. Still, they reasoned, a patient could not possibly be harmed by large doses of vitamin E since the body would simply discard what it did not need. So why not try another experiment?

Their second patient was Dr. Shute's own mother, seventy-one years old, who suffered from angina pectoris. To avoid bringing on the agonizing pains of this heart disease, she was forced to avoid all exercise.

Also, her arms and legs were waterlogged from excess fluids in the tissues. Vitamin E was given to her in the same large, highly concentrated doses as had been tried on the old man in the hospital. After five days the pain had disappeared from her chest and the swelling had subsided from her limbs.

Since their discovery, these three doctors have treated some 4,000 heart patients with this vitamin. Nor do they confine the treatment to any one type of heart disease. Hypertensive heart disease, coronary occlusion, rheumatic heart disease, angina pectoris, heart tissue starvation resulting from hardening of the arteries all these forms of grave heart disorders have been treated with vitamin E.

Of 84 patients suffering the pains of angina pectoris, 52 per cent were completely relieved, and 44 percent showed some improvement. In 28 cases of rheumatic heart disease, 53 percent showed marked betterment, and 43 percent were relieved somewhat.

In 65 cases of high blood pressure (hypertension), 42 percent showed remarkable improvement, while 43 percent received some relief. Dramatic results were obtained with one man, a wheel-chair invalid. So advanced was his case of heart disease that even prolonged conversation would bring on an acute attack of angina pectoris.

But after treatment with large doses of highly concentrated vitamin E, this patient left his wheel chair. He reported having fished all day, and then played bridge until midnight. And next day he played nine holes of golf.

Another patient, a twenty six year old man, had been incapacitated since an attack of rheumatic fever suffered in childhood. After being treated with vitamin E, this man obtained employment in a foundry where he was reported on the job every day.

Still another patient, seventy-one years old, had been laid up for years because of angina pectoris which would attack him at the slightest exertion. After his treatment, he went to work in a tannery, performing heavy labor!

Dr. Wilfred Shute, basing his statement on the astonishing results obtained, says that vitamin E is the most effective known "drug" in the treatment of heart disease, and certainly the safest.

Dr. Evan Shute's summing up of the case of vitamin E is one of the most forthright statements to come from the medical profession in years. It is hard to imagine, says Dr. Shute that what vitamin E does to clots in superficial blood vessels it cannot also do for the vessels of the heart. However, he continues, the controversy can be settled with ease.

All that is necessary is for an unprejudiced cardiac clinic to treat alternate patients with vitamin E and with traditional remedies. The results, predicts Dr. Shute, will tell the story quickly, for "if we are wrong, it will be simple to prove it, and if we are right, everyone should know about it."

Vitamin E has also proved remarkably effective in treating other diseased conditions of the body brought on by an insufficient blood supply, such as thrombosis and phlebitis, chronic leg ulcers, Buerger's disease and even gangrene in early stages.

It should be noted that the vitamin E given by Drs. Shute and Dr. Vogelsang is in capsule form, to be taken by mouth. I make this point to clear up any misunderstanding that might arise in the minds of readers that it would be necessary to submit to a pro-longed series of expensive injections.

Further, the capsules should contain not less than 30 International Units of vitamin E. The common vitamin E capsules containing wheat germ oil are not highly concentrated enough to have the desired effect on the heart, since they contain comparatively negligible amounts of vitamin E. And so, in speaking of vitamin E for treating the heart, it is understood that reference is made to the new highly concentrated capsules recently developed.

Ordinarily vitamin E is the commonest of all vitamins, being present in the germ of all grains, in leafy and root vegetables, and in meat.

At first glance, it would seem that a person eating a balanced diet would obtain enough vitamin E from his food to ward off, or to relieve, heart disease. Why, then, must heart disease be prevented, or relieved, by highly concentrated doses of a vitamin that appears or should appear in every daily diet?

The answer is that our "civilized" menus have been systematically purged of a normal quantity of this vitamin. The white bread on our tables, even most of the so-called "whole wheat" bread, retains only a trace of its normal vitamin E content; the vitamin E in fruit is present in the peel and the core, both of which are seldom consumed; in root vegetables (potatoes, beets, turnips) most of the vitamin E is in the skin which is removed before these vegetables find their way to our plates; in leafy vegetables, the greater part of vitamin E is found in the coarse outer leaves, and rarely are these used by our cooks.

I agree wholeheartedly with certain medical scientists who claim that we are more deficient in vitamin E than in any other vitamin, thanks to our "refined" food tastes.

This tragic lack of a vitamin that nature intended us to consume in liberal quantities undoubtedly has great bearing on the alarming increase in circulatory disorders among us.

As proof of this link between vitamin E starvation and cardiac disease, we know that primitive peoples are almost complete strangers to heart ailments until they begin eating our civilized food. Then the Eskimo, the Indian or the Polynesian contracts heart ailments as readily as his white brother.

Chapter 5

Food Supplements

Besides vitamin E, other food supplements have proved their worth in treating heart disorders. Vitamin B-complex, containing thiamin, is prescribed by many physicians for their heart patients. Dr. Robert S. Bergh off, eminent Chicago heart specialist, says that thiamin (vitamin B-1) is of definite value in the treatment of coronary heart trouble.

The minerals calcium and phosphorus nourish and soothe the starving, irritable heart nerves, and certainly these two minerals should not be overlooked by anyone desirous of maintaining a healthy heart, or calming a heart that is plagued by over excitability.

The mineral potassium, too, has been found by a group of Philadelphia doctors to be needed by a healthy heart. Severe cases of diabetes, with consequent vomiting and serious diarrhea, showed a changed heart action, as recorded by the electro-cardiogram, owing to the body's depletion of potassium.

However, when potassium was given to the patients, the heart reading became more nearly normal, and the patients improved. These, then, are the food supplements which we know exert beneficial effects on the heart, either relieving its ailments or pre-venting it from developing harmful or annoying disturbances: Vitamin E, vitamin B-complex (containing thiamin), and the minerals calcium, phosphorus and potassium.

What should the heart patient eat? Diet is as vital to a heart patient's welfare as to that of a diabetic.

Chapter 6

The Heart Patient

The first important topic is the foods the heart patient should not eat. He must stay away from all gas-producing or hard to digest foods. I say this because such foods cause the digestive organs (most of which are next-door neighbors to the heart) to bloat and crowd against the heart.

This, in itself, is enough to bring on an attack of angina. While each patient must note for himself what is hard to digest, practically everyone finds all vegetables of the cabbage family (cauliflower, Brussels sprouts, broccoli), as well as onions, and dried beans and peas to be gas-producing.

Sweet potatoes and yellow squash also cause gas to form within the digestive tract. This holds true also of foods such as highly seasoned sauces and gravies, and rich desserts, particularly those containing chocolate.

Salt, too, is taboo in the diet of the heart patient. Aside from the damage which ordinary table salt can do to the kidneys and the arteries, the heart patient must consider the abnormal thirst which highly salted foods produce.

Formerly the heart patient was restricted as to the amount of fluids he could take. But it has been found that a low salt diet keeps thirst under control, and the patient does not need to curtail a normal consumption of liquids.

However, strong tea or coffee, as well as excessive alcohol, can do a diseased or an exhausted heart nothing but harm.

Low Salt Diet

A low salt diet as prescribed for the heart patient should not include such items as canned soups, vegetables, fish or meat; pickles; olives; prepared salad dressing; gelatin desserts; milk (lactic acid tablets are a good substitute); soda fountain drinks; salty crackers or biscuits. Incidentally, as a sweetening agent, there is no finer food than honey to replace the "refined" sugars, be they white, tan or brown.

Chapter 7

Miracle Honey

Honey is a pre-digested food easily converted by the human digestive organs into the type of sugars utilized by the heart muscle for energy. When to eat is almost as important to the heart patient as what to eat. Four or five light meals a day are far safer than three heavy meals, since there is far less danger of overburdening the heart by making it supply enormous quantities of blood to the digestive organs so they can process heavy meals.

Also, the light meals will avoid distending the stomach and crowding it against the heart. The most substantial meal should be eaten in the middle of the day, and no meal should be taken later than four hours before bedtime, although a cup of herb tea may be drunk shortly before retiring to appease the stomach if there is a sensation of hunger at this time.

Moreover, the heart patient who is overweight should restrict his diet to 1,200 calories per day. Any patient in bed, or whose exercise is curtailed, does not need more than 1,800 calories per day, while those on moderate activity do best on 2,400 calories.

I want to emphasize that a major portion of all these diets for the heart patient, regardless of their caloric value, should be composed of high protein foods.

This is essential, since protein is the tissue building food element, and certainly the heart tissues, as well as all others throughout the body, must constantly be repaired and restored if the patient is to respond well to other treatment.

I shall dwell more at length on the need for protein in the diet in a later chapter, but I do want to give this advice to those persons suffering from heart ailments: Make sure you eat enough of the high-protein foods such as broiled or roasted meat, natural cheese or eggs.

If, for some reason, these foods cannot be tolerated, then the diet should be supplemented with concentrated amino acids to make certain that sufficient protein is supplied so the body tissues can be kept in good repair. However you get it, don't neglect protein!

Chronic constipation (often resulting from improperly chosen diets) is a serious aggravation to a heart suffering from any type of disorder. Do not add insult to injury by forcing a weakened or a tired heart to maintain life in a body clogged with poisonous wastes.

I should not have to remind anyone that harsh laxatives compounded of synthetic drugs are by no means to be considered the answer to the constipation problem.

And so I have mention some of the foods that can cause heart trouble true and false; I have pointed out to you the incalculable damage that unbridled thinking can cause the heart; I have reported to you the promising new method of treating heart disorders with highly concentrated vitamin E; and I have outlined what the diet should and should not be for the heart sufferer.

The rest is up to you. We have it within our own power to prevent, heal or alleviate our own heart disturbances by a calm acceptance of our condition, an earnest determination to keep the mind free from all irritations and fears, and by faithful adherence to prove diets and therapeutic treatments. Your heart is in your own hands!

Rossie C Pattison

Chapter 8

Why the Health of the Red Blood Cells Are Vital

Anemics are only half-alive

Good red blood has the power to create vigorous health in the human body. An anemic body is a half-starved vessel crying out for more and more of the vital fluids imperative to its existence.

Rain penetrates below the surface of the ground, combining with the soil-contained minerals to produce plant food in liquid, readily assimilable form so that plant roots may drink deep and partake of the earth's nourishment.

49

Like rain, blood is a liquid; it flows into the body tissues, bringing food in the form of oxygen that has been picked up in the lungs, as well as other nutritive substances (minerals, amino acids, hormones and vitamins) that have entered the bloodstream through the intestinal walls or by direct secretion of certain endocrine glands.

Even as plant roots cannot make use of the mineral food in the soil until it is put into solution by ground moisture, so the body cannot use the oxygen we breathe, or the food we eat, until it reaches the bloodstream where it is conveyed, in solution, to the hungry body cells.

That very solid-looking piece of roast beef you ate for dinner will have to be converted into highly soluble protein (amino acids) before it can feed your tired muscles.

That substance called "air," which we breathe, but cannot see, must have its oxygen extracted by the lungs and delivered over to the hemoglobin ring in the red blood cells before that oxygen can revitalize the trillions of body cells.

Blood can be described, therefore, in brief as the conveyor system by means of which nourishment, extracted from the "raw materials" provided by the lungs and digestive tract, reaches the hungry body cells.

Unless this blood conveyor system is operating at top efficiency, the body cannot remain in good working order any more than a stalk of wheat will thrive in parched earth.

When it happens as it so often does that the human blood system is not operating at maximum efficiency, we say that a person has anemia. Anemia itself is not a killer disease, but it is the number one cause why so many persons seem only half-alive. Anemia lets down the bars of body resistance, inviting serious infections to enter. Anyone may become anemic, at any time.

Most persons either have had, or will have, anemia at some time in their lives. Anemia among younger persons is usually not difficult to overcome. But in anyone over forty, anemia offers a more serious problem. During and after this period of life, a diagnosis of "anemia" should call for immediate action.

Anemia is an insidious ailment that can fasten upon us without giving any drastic warning signals. Anemia is a vitality thief. It robs the body of the energy needed for vigorous living.

There is no doubt in my mind that the majority of patients suffering from diseases brought on by their emotionally underpar minds will also be found to be anywhere from slightly to seriously anemic; for how can half-fed brain cells contribute to keen, logical thinking?

Brains cells that are to generate strong, healthy thoughts must be nourished constantly by a flow of blood that contains plenty of red blood cells charged to the utmost with hemoglobin, the oxygen carrier.

The tragic thing about anemic blood is that it is so wasteful. A person suffering from anemia may eat adequate, well-balanced meals, and yet be slowly starving his body cells merely because his blood is not equipped with sufficient food conveyors (red blood cells) to pick up and carry the nourishment for which the hungry cells are pleading.

And so a good portion of the nourishment that ordinarily would find its way to the cells is lost from the body in the faces and in the urine, all because there are not enough red blood cell conveyors to deliver the food to its intended destination within the trillions of body cells.

This wasteful situation is similar to that which would exist in a city if food were to arrive in the wholesale markets when there were not enough trucks and drivers to see that the supplies were widely distributed throughout every neighborhood. The city's people would go hungry in the midst of plenty. And so it is with the body cells in an anemic body they are literally ravenous in the midst of a feast!

Before going any further, I want to dispel one current misconception about anemia: Not always is it the thin, sallow, run-down person who is anemic, since a majority of overweight persons are anywhere from slightly too seriously anemic. In fact, it is their anemia that keeps them always hungry, always eating more and more in an effort to assuage that craving for food. And instead of being utilized by the cells as it should, the food is piled up as fat in different parts of the body.

Chapter 9

Obesity

Numerous cases of obesity have cleared up like magic when first the anemia was overcome so the patient's bloodstream could carry a maximum of nourishment to the body cells with a minimum intake of food calories. To understand how anemia is caused, let's take a quick look at the ingredients of that miracle fluid blood.

If scientists were able to make blood in the laboratory, they would need plasma, red blood cells and white blood cells as the basis for this fluid of life. Plasma is the salty, straw-colored liquid in which floats the red and white blood cells, together with the nutritive substances absorbed through the intestinal walls, or the hormones deposited directly in the bloodstream by certain glands. About one gallon of this plasma or "blood water" is contained in the blood vessels of the body.

The red blood cells swimming around in this gallon of salt water are something like 24 billion, and they are so tiny that 3,000 of them placed in a row would measure barely one inch! The white blood cells are only 1/1000th as numerous as the red blood cells. (When these white blood cells, intended by nature to protect the bloodstream from bacteria invaders, multiply out of all proportion, they cause that often fatal disease known as leukemia, often called "blood cancer.")

The leading character of this drama entitled "Fluid of Life" is the red blood cell, truly a temperamental fellow. If he doesn't get what he likes to eat, he walks offstage and refuses to perform. Equally as serious, he shows no interest in the future generations of his kind. Whether the body cells get oxygen or whether new red blood cells are born to take his place at the end of his life-span of thirty to ninety days is none of his worry.

Let the blood become anemic, he says with a shrug; it's all the same to him if the owner of that blood isn't interested enough in the body's health to see that the red blood cells get the particular delicacies that delight their cellular appetites! This temperamental fellow, the red blood cell, is created within the bone marrow. He is not exactly a "glamour" cell in looks, being nothing but a tiny flat disc with a small depression in the center on both sides. Roughly, the red blood cell resembles a doughnut, except that the center is a depression rather than a hole.

The outer ring around this depressed center is where the red blood cell wears his hemoglobin. It is this pigment, hemoglobin, that gives the red blood cell his glowing, crimson color so famed in poem and story. Without hemoglobin, the red blood cell is indeed a pale, colorless, washed out fellow about as pallid as the anemic person who does not have enough red blood cells!

If we are to tell the complete story of the red blood cell, we must confess that he is merely the container designed by nature to hold the bloodstream's supply of hemoglobin within the meshes of that sponge-like outer ring of his doughnut-shaped cell.

Strictly speaking, hemoglobin is the real star of the blood drama, rather than the red blood cell himself, since the red blood cell is rather like the supers in the pageant of opera who bear the tenor across the stage on their shoulders. Although the red blood cells, like the supers, do manage to get on stage, yet their entry does not contribute much to the scene if hemoglobin does not appear.

But hemoglobin, too, carries something vital to the drama, just as the tenor in opera may bear in his hand a stage prop such as a knife or a scroll necessary to further the action of the plot. The prop that hemoglobin carries is oxygen when it enters the scene (tissue cells), and carbon dioxide when it exits via the veins.

Chapter 10

Hemoglobin

Hemoglobin, the red pigment, is a complex chemical substance with a high capacity for absorbing oxygen while in the lungs, and with the further valuable trait of being able to exchange that oxygen in the tissues for the waste product, carbon dioxide, which it brings back to the lungs to be expelled in the outgoing breath.

Although oxygen is vital to the health of all other body cells, the red blood cell itself consumes no appreciable part of the oxygen it is carrying. The explanation for this is that the red blood cell in the bloodstream is not a living cell; it is alive and in need of oxygen only while going through the creative and growing process within the bone marrow.

When the red blood cell is finally mature enough to be launched from the bone marrow into the bloodstream, it is like a ship, already built, designed to last a certain time, then to be withdrawn from active service at the end of that period.

As we have said, the average life span of a red blood cell is from thirty to ninety days. At the end of this period, after the red blood cell has become too decrepit to keep up with the crowd, or when it has been imperfectly formed, certain star-shaped cells in the liver reach out with their tentacles to drag the worn-out or deformed red blood cell out of the swim.

And, because Dame Nature can be a thrifty as well as a prodigal housekeeper, she sees to it that the hemoglobin of the old or misshapen red blood cells does not go to waste.

Chapter 11

Anemia Diet and Nutrition

The star-cells of the liver extract the hemoglobin from the junked red blood cells, funneling a portion of it through the liver to be used in making the green bile pigment, while the balance of the discarded hemoglobin is converted into a hormone that helps stimulate the formation of new red blood cells within the bone marrow.

Within this bone-marrow factory, the red blood cell demands a diet entirely to his liking. This diet for the growing red blood cell is four-fold with the fourth substance remaining, as yet, more or less of a mystery to the hematologists (blood scientists), although there is great hope that they have hit upon it in the newly discovered vitamin B-12.

60

The three other food elements in this rigidly prescribed diet for the growing and multiplying red blood cell are common substances contained in every normal, adequate diet: protein (amino acids), vitamins (especially C and the B-complex group), together with the organic minerals copper and iron.

Our principal concern at this moment is with iron, because this mineral is the key factor in determining whether blood is healthy or anemic. In fact, the common type of nutritional anemia is called iron-deficiency anemia to distinguish it from pernicious anemia, a disease of an entirely different character.

Hemoglobin, when analyzed in the laboratory, is found to contain iron as its essential and principal ingredient. When the blood plasma contains far too few red blood cells, or when the red blood cells it does contain are "more hole than doughnut," that is, more center depression than hemoglobin ring, then a person is said to be suffering from iron-deficiency anemia.

Looking at a drop of normal blood under a powerful microscope, we would see a thick population of red blood cells with plump, oxygen filled outer rims of hemoglobin. A drop of slightly anemic blood would show approximately one-third less red blood cells in the group, and these cells would show evidences of narrower rims of hemoglobin.

A drop of seriously anemic blood would have about one-half the number of red blood cells that should be contained in healthy blood; and the cells that were present would be mere shadows of their "hemoglobin selves," since the outer rim of this oxygen-carrying red pigment would be a mere tracing.

Therefore, anemic blood means not only fewer red blood cells than normal, but also the presence of red blood cells woefully lacking in hemoglobin.

Anemia brings not only a decrease in the quantity of red blood cells, but also a falling off in the quality of those cells, that is, in their ability to carry oxygen. In an anemic body, the bone marrow (where the red blood cells are created) is like a factory that works only part time, turning out fewer and fewer products of poorer and poorer quality.

The one way to turn that run down bone marrow factory into an efficient plant is to make sure that plenty of iron is on hand to assure the processing of a full quota of high-grade red blood cells containing a maximum of hemoglobin.

Iron is the master builder of hemoglobin in the blood; iron is the body's master mineral because it creates warmth, vitality, stamina. With plenty of usable iron in the blood, we are more likely to be vigorous in every sense of the word. Why should the iron content in anyone's blood fall below normal? Failing to include sufficient iron-rich foods in the diet will cause the body to draw upon its iron reserves until a dangerously low level is reached. Meat particularly beefs liver and kidneys, dark poultry meat, and lean beef are especially rich in iron.

The high price of meat during me early postwar years caused many families unknowingly to invite that unwelcome guest, anemia, into their midst all because they could not afford to serve regular and plentiful portions of this iron-rich food.

Physicians noted a sharp rise in the number of their anemia patients, beginning with World War II days when meat was severely rationed and continuing through the postwar era of high-cost meat products.

Then there are the persons mostly women who actually inflict themselves with anemia in a misguided effort to get slim, or to remain so, by munching on nothing heartier than salads and dainty sandwiches. Women are more vulnerable to the onset of anemia than men, since they require three to four times as much iron as men during a lifetime in order to replace the valuable supplies of body iron lost through menstruation and pregnancy.

For a woman who is constantly losing iron through the menstrual flow to deplete further her body reserves of iron by subsisting on a sandwich salad diet is nothing short of health suicide! The principal reason why I frown on a strictly vegetarian diet is because it cannot possibly supply adequate quantities of iron or protein to maintain maximum health and vitality. I am not attempting to convert the confirmed vegetarians.

Yet I do urge them to supplement their diets with mineral iron and with protein in the form of concentrated amino acids if they wish to avoid the numerous deficiency diseases, particularly anemia.

Chapter 12

Inexpensive Way to Obtain More Iron in Your Diet

A good, inexpensive way to obtain extra iron may be prepared at home. Buy some unsulphured apricots (usually found only in health food stores); or, if apricots are not available, the next best in order are dried peaches, then raisins. Put a handful of the fruit in the bottom of a drinking glass, cover with lukewarm water, stir, and let stand overnight. The next morning stir the mixture again; pour the water into another glass, adding a tablespoonful of unsulphured molasses. Prepare and drink this several times a week. The fruit, of course, may also be used. This "tonic," however, is intended only to supplement, not to replace, the iron-rich foods necessary to every well-balanced diet.

Anemia is also likely to afflict those persons who have been forced to adhere to a strict diet because of some diseased condition of the gastro-intestinal tract or the kidneys. These persons should supplement their diets with iron, perhaps in tablet form, if it is found this is the way they can best tolerate the supplement.

Occasionally we find an anemia patient whose ailment persists despite a conscientious effort to supply the body with plenty of iron-rich foods. The trouble here is that the iron cannot be absorbed into the bloodstream because the stomach fails to produce enough hydrochloric acid to convert the iron into readily assimilable form.

Or it may be that hemorrhaging in some part of the body is depleting the iron reserves faster than they can be replenished through ordinary diet. This can happen if blood continually seeps from unhealthy gums. Perhaps the fault may also lie with bleeding ulcers, or with hemorrhoids. In women, the cause may be traced to the presence of fibroid tumors or to some menstrual disturbance.

Chronic diarrhea, too, will interfere with proper absorption of iron into the bloodstream, since the intestines will be forced to hurry along their contents before the vitally needed food elements can be extracted and passed through the intestinal walls into the bloodstream.

And, too, the presence of parasites in the intestines can cause anemia by withdrawing blood from the mucous lining of the intestinal walls more rapidly than it can be replaced. Cirrhosis of the liver, when chronic, will also interfere with this organ's ability to store the iron and other nutritive elements needed to prevent anemia.

Infections of long standing in the body may bring on anemia because of the contamination they introduce into the bloodstream, thereby threatening the production of healthy red blood cells in the bone marrow. Nor should we overlook the fact that anemia often results when certain chemical poisons invade the bone marrow where the fate of the red blood cell is determined. Although this may happen in the case of workers in a chemical factory, the most likely cause is in the continued use of strong chemical medicines.

Chapter 13

How Can You Tell Whether Or Not You Are Anemic?

Fatigue is the most prominent symptom of iron-deficiency anemia. A chronic, low-grade tiredness that persists regardless of adequate rest and relaxation is almost certain to be a warning of anemia. When the body tissues are short of oxygen, weakness, lassitude and abnormal fatigue set in rather quickly. This is logical when we remember that anemic blood does not have enough red blood cells with high haemoglobin carrying power to supply the body tissues with sufficient oxygen or to pick up from the cells the waste product, carbon dioxide.

68

Thus the tissue cells in an anemic body are both hungry and polluted. Is it any wonder, then, that the entire body should be weak, tired and wholly unequal to meet the demands of normal living? Persons with anemia of long duration often experience changes in their facial expression, as well as in the color of the complexion, to say nothing of their hopeless mental attitude! The countenance assumes a look of utter dejection and hopelessness, mirroring the general condition of mind and body.

Naturally the mental attitude of such persons will be at a low ebb, the same as their physical resistance, since hungry, waste-polluted brain cells can no more remain healthy than the cells of the nervous system or the tissue cells in the muscles or other vital organs.

A seriously anemic person is often too tired mentally to make wise decisions or to formulate plans with keen perception. Further, the mind of an anemic person is often so weary that small happenings have a habit of magnifying themselves into major incidents. Brooding over failure or personal inadequacies is common in minds not clicking one hundred percent because the brain cells are inadequately served by anemic blood.

And, of course, the longer the anemia continues, the more fixed becomes the pattern of brooding and emotional imagining, with the result that the groundwork is often laid for the onset of mind-induced illnesses.

An employer once told me that, if such a thing were possible, he would make it a rule that no seriously anemic person would be allowed to work in his office.

Why? Because it was his experience that anemic persons not only were incapable of efficient workmanship and clear thinking, but they also tended to be overly sensitive to a point where a friendly correction was magnified by them into the crudest rebuke! Especially does anemia seem to fasten onto women men, too during the climacteric (change of life), perhaps because of some glandular disruption. During this period of change and readjustment, the endocrine glands are susceptible to over- or under-stimulation.

If you suspect the presence of anemia at any age, and especially after forty, do not shrug it off as something "not very serious," for anemia after forty is an ailment that can shorten your years of useful, vigorous living. And certainly the mind of anyone suffering with anemia is not equipped to cope with the bewildering personal adjustments that must be faced and accepted after the fourth decade.

Chapter 14

Symptoms of Anemia

Symptoms of anemia do not appear, as a rule, until after the hemoglobin content and the number of red blood cells have been reduced appreciably. The fatigue and loss of vigor that accompany anemia do not make a sudden appearance; they set in gradually, wearing away the body's vitality and mental reserves. So insidiously does anemia sneak up on its victim that the first feeling of unexplainable weariness turns into utter exhaustion almost before the victim is aware of what has happened.

The fingernails and toenails become tender, flattened, indented or brittle; the hair is dry and becomes lusterless, often turning prematurely gray; the skin, too, loses its youthful freshness,

71

wrinkling easily. These symptoms of anemia appear early in the disorder, since iron is stored principally in the hair, skin and nails.

And when not enough iron is provided in the diet, the bone marrow begins to draw on the reserve stocks for creation of new blood cells, with the result that the structure of the hair, skin and nails changes drastically as the continued withdrawal of reserve iron leaves them more and more depleted.

The mouth and tongue, too, show the effects of anemic blood. The mouth is likely to feel sore and tender; the tongue burns, becoming unusually slick and smooth, and often beefy red in color. As the number of red blood cells grows fewer and fewer, containing less and less hemoglobin, the victim of anemia shows increasing evidence of this weaker, paler blood that is gradually starving his entire body. His skin becomes pasty white, especially that in the ear lobes and the whites of his eyes assume a blue-white hue.

Shortness of breath and palpitation of the heart usually appear when the blood is too poor in hemoglobin to nourish and cleanse the heart muscle properly. Like the skin, the hair, the brain cells and the other vital organs, the heart cannot remain healthy when the red blood cells that are supposed to feed it and to carry away its waste products are not only pitifully few in numbers but also seriously lacking in hemoglobin.

The heart, like any other muscle, will begin to show signs of the strain of continuing to function under adverse conditions. The slightest exertion will cause the victim of anemia to pant and puff. Or the heart may flutter and "flop" for no apparent reason.

Frequently these heart symptoms will disappear as soon as the blood is built up to its normal consistency. Anyone who is bothered by shortness of breath, dizziness, or a palpitating heart should have a thorough examination of that organ by a competent physician. And if he pronounces the heart "O.K." despite these annoying symptoms, the next thing to suspect is anemia.

Here is an important word of warning: Even though the heart may have shown no signs of damage at the first examination, unless anemia is checked as rapidly as possible, the heart will suffer ultimate damage. Further, I foresee the day when hematologists will discover that anemic blood tends to sludge more readily than healthy, iron-rich blood. We have seen in the previous chapter that sludged blood is a menace not only to maximum health, but to life itself.

Therefore, anemia not only robs the body of health and vigor, but it also prepares the way for more serious, often fatal, diseases. Anemia is more than mere "tiredness"; it is the tragic evidence that body cells are starved and waste-polluted because the red blood cells have fallen down on the job.

Any humane person would hasten to relieve the wretchedness of a helpless, bed-ridden fellow being, half-dead from malnutrition. Certainly what we would do for another person should be no more than we would do for our own bodies. Each cell in an anemic body is comparable to the helpless patient, dying of starvation amid accumulating wastes.

Chapter 15

Restoring the Blood to Normal

If the blood is anemic for the simple reason that the body lacks sufficient iron to create enough red blood cells with plenty of hemoglobin, then the remedy likewise is a simple one: More iron taken by mouth in the form of a tonic or in tablets, in addition to a diet rich in vitamins and high-grade protein foods. After several weeks the blood can be built up to normal under this treatment. The hemoglobin should rise at least 1 percent each day. When the blood has become less anemic, the patient starts noticing that his endurance and vitality have increased accordingly not to mention his enthusiasm for living and his ability to think more clearly!

However, if merely supplementing the diet with iron does not bring results after a few weeks, the patient should undergo a thorough physical examination to determine what bodily condition might be responsible for the continuing anemia.

In other words, to find out what is interfering with the creation of more and healthier red blood cells despite the fact that the necessary ingredient, iron, is bountifully supplied. But by no means should the iron supplements be discontinued, for to do so would be to aggravate further an already serious condition.

No discussion of anemia and its treatment would be complete without mentioning chlorophyll, the substance that makes plant blood green, just as hemoglobin makes animal blood red. Science has been amazed to discover that chlorophyll bears a striking chemical resemblance to the hemoglobin of human blood.

Thus it is only natural that chlorophyll should have suggested itself as a treatment for anemia. This green plant blood, in tablet form, was given by several medical researchers to anemia patients who responded by showing increased hemoglobin content in the blood within a remarkably short time. Chlorophyll, being a natural substance, is not a drug; it is non-toxic, and produces no unfavorable reactions.

Dr. Boris Berkman, an eminent scientist, reported not long ago that he believed chlorophyll might be used successfully to help stave off the ravages of age.

He said further that chlorophyll might help overcome the slowing down of oxidation (making use of the oxygen brought by the red blood cells) with the advance of old age, thereby helping combat the degenerative diseases of later years such as anemia, and hardening of the arteries.

The therapeutic values of chlorophyll are such that this "plant hemoglobin" deserves wider use among anemia sufferers than it has as yet achieved, perhaps because the mineral iron has overshadowed its properties.

But there is some evidence to prove that chlorophyll, taken in conjunction with iron, promotes the efficiency of this mineral in controlling or preventing anemia.

Up to this point we have been speaking exclusively of the symptoms and treatment of simple iron-deficiency anemia which comprises about 95 percent of all anemia cases.

However, there is another type of blood disorder called pernicious anemia. Up until about twenty years ago, pernicious anemia was inevitably fatal. Even now, unless diagnosed during its early stages and treated immediately, pernicious anemia can be a killer disease. It attacks not only the blood, but also the mouth, the stomach and, most serious of all, the central nervous system.

The Vitamin B12 Solution

Chapter 16

Pernicious Anemia

Pernicious anemia, therefore, involves more than a blood disorder. If this serious disease is allowed to progress, certain nerves in the spine degenerate, bringing on paralysis of the arms and legs, and in some instances a disturbed mental condition.

For some reason, as yet not known to us, pernicious anemia seldom develops until after the age of thirty, and its victims are most likely to be inhabitants of the United States, Canada and Northern Europe. Although we hesitate to say definitely that pernicious anemia is hereditary, we do know that it is frequently found in certain families.

The symptoms of pernicious anemia in the early stages resemble those of iron-deficiency anemia. Easy, unexplainable fatigue is the outstanding characteristic of early pernicious anemia; the least exertion may cause breathlessness and heart palpitations. In some patients, the ankles will swell. All desire for food departs; often the mere sight of a meal may cause nausea. In fact, nausea and vomiting are not unusual.

The hands and feet may tingle and grow numb to such an extent that the victim is greatly distressed. The mouth and tongue suffer intermittent attacks of soreness when the tongue becomes smooth and so red it looks as though it had been seared with a hot iron.

The typical victim of pernicious anemia is often prematurely gray, with a skin so bloodless and pallid that it actually looks lemon yellow. The most important thing I can impress upon you about pernicious anemia is the vital need for early diagnosis. This is a killer disease that must be detected and controlled as quickly as possible.

Like diabetes, there is no cure for pernicious anemia, but it can be controlled and lived with to a ripe old age, thanks to liver. In other words, liver extract is the "insulin" of the pernicious anemia patient. Without it, he must surely waste away and die; with liver, he can live a long, useful, comparatively comfortable life.

Several years ago, folic acid burst upon the scene as the "white hope" of pernicious anemia sufferers. It seemed quite possible that folic acid would obviate the need for continuous injections of liver extract (this type of anemia does not respond well to food liver or liver extract taken by mouth).

Folic acid did prove to be a remarkable stimulant to the production of normal blood, although it was not able to check degeneration of the central nervous system. Only concentrated liver extract, up to the present time, is able to perform this vital function for the victim of pernicious anemia.

But folic acid is a very valuable blood-building vitamin found in the B-complex group, and most certainly can be used, in conjunction with mineral iron and chlorophyll, to overcome simple anemia, and to help control pernicious anemia as a supplement to liver injections.

We have long known that a member of the vitamin B-complex group was an indispensable aide-de-camp to iron in preventing and overcoming simple nutritional anemia. But not until a few years ago did we isolate that substance and call it folic acid (because it was found in the foliage of spinach).

Although folic acid is not a substitute for ample diets rich in iron and protein, this member of the vitamin B-complex group has earned a permanent place as an adjunct in the treatment of both simple and pernicious anemia by its wonderful power to stimulate the bone marrow into turning out more normal quantities of healthy red blood cells.

Rossie C Pattison

Vitamin B-12

Promising news for all anemia victims comes from the research laboratories in the announcement that vitamin B-12 has been isolated from liver. This newest vitamin is seen as red, needle like crystals.

The important thing about the new vitamin B-12 when and if it becomes plentiful enough to supply the market is that it promises to release the victim of pernicious anemia from the unceasing need for expensive liver injections.

A single dose of 3 micro-grams of the new crystalline B-12 (barely enough to cover the head of a pin) was sufficient to give positive results when tested on three pernicious anemia patients by Dr. West of the Department of Medicine, Columbia University.

Comparing the new vitamin B-12 with the usual concentrated liver extract, the laboratories estimate that the ability of this new vitamin to fight anemia is at least a million times more potent than the present liver injections!

Meanwhile, until vitamin B-12 has been more widely tested and has been produced in a form that will be within reach of the pocket-books of all anemia victims, my best advice to those afflicted with both simple anemia and pernicious anemia is this: Keep up present treatments of iron, chlorophyll, folic acid or liver extract.

Make sure the diet contains ample servings of meats such as liver, sweetbreads and kidneys, varied with red meats trimmed of all fat. Include in the diet fresh fruits and green vegetables, along with whole grain cereals and apricots. Salt and fats should be used only sparingly.

Incidentally, for anyone who is unable to tolerate liver served rare, I suggest grinding it fine, and serving in tomato juice or soup. The thought occurs to me that there may be a very good reason why anemia, and especially pernicious anemia, strikes almost exclusively the peoples of the United States, Canada and Northern Europe.

It is in these countries that the people confine their meat dishes principally to the lean muscle tissues, discarding the iron rich parts such as the heart, kidneys, liver, lungs, and sweetbreads. Farther south in Europe, the traveler finds these meats, so ill-favored in the north, gracing the tables of rich and poor alike.

In fact, like primitive tribes, the Southern European considers these internal organs a great delicacy and has devised tasty ways of serving them. Perhaps we should legislate for a return to an old custom that was prevalent in Europe during the middle ages. Children of that day were obliged to eat bread made from whole grain dough mixed with ground liver.

Whatever may have been the diseases that carried off the young in that unhygienic era, certainly anemia was not one of them! Could it be that our passion for white bread and beefsteak is responsible for the anemia that threatens to attack, in more or less serious form, every American at some stage of his life?

Truly, "the life of the flesh is in the blood". Take care of your red blood cells, and your hemoglobin will take care of you physically and mentally!

Chapter 17

The Body Cells

Sludged Blood is a term you will probably be hearing more and more about in the days to come. Sludged blood may even be the missing link in the study of mind body diseases. We know that poorly nourished brain cells mean uncontrolled mental processes and poor emotional control means trouble for the rest of the body. But why and how this vicious chain of reactions takes place, we have been able only to guess until lately when the results of a seventeen-year study of human blood were made known.

Medical research has discovered that human blood can form sludge as thick and as injurious as any engine sludge that ever clogged the lubrication system of an automobile.

The word "sludge" is applied to any thick, non-fluid matter that forms in an otherwise free flowing medium. The harmful, corrosive sediment found in a steam boiler is spoken of as "sludge"; the solid matter that results from sewage treatment processes is also known as "sludge."

In other words, sludge is an unwelcome product. And now science has discovered that human blood (as well as the blood of lesser animals) can form sludge as harmful and as un-wanted as any sludge that complicates the operation of a piece of machinery.

For centuries, philosophers and scientists have attempted to uncover the secret of life. Although the brilliant French physician and philosopher, Dr. Carrel, did succeed in keeping a piece of chicken heart alive since 1912, the true secret of life has never been revealed to our learned scientists.

But now we have probed into the inner secrets of that equally mystifying state, death, and for the first time in all the long history of medical science, we know why death comes.

Specially constructed cameras have photographed the startling changes that take place in the blood of a dying animal. The lens has recorded the dramatic sequence of death from its onset until the final moment. We note the gradual thickening of the blood until the fatal moment when the great amount of sludge clogging the blood vessels causes circulation to cease entirely.

Chapter 18

Why Sludged Blood Causes the Human Body to Deteriorate

Discovery of how and why sludged blood causes the human body to deteriorate gradually, then finally die will make it possible for thousands of persons to add years of useful living to their "allotted span" of days. Knowledge of the injurious effect sludged blood has on the human mind and nervous system will make it possible for thousands more persons to clear up their foggy thinking and to calm their jittery nerves either by taking care to see that their blood does not become sludged, or by hastening to remove the sludge already formed in the arteries.

The relationship between psychosomatic (mind-induced) diseases and blood sludge is only beginning to be suspected. Yet the conclusion is quite evident that brain tissue improperly nourished because the blood cannot flow freely and rapidly throughout the vast labyrinth of brain cells will be brain tissue unequal to meet the demands of an active, healthy mind!

Sludged blood can cause the central nervous system which includes the brain to become so underpar that the groundwork is laid for the so called "psychosomatic" illnesses. Exactly how does this blood sludge form and why does it cause so much damage that death is inevitable over a varying period of time? Before answering this question, let's have a quick review of the human circulatory system for those who may have forgotten their physiology:

Blood (freshly oxygenated and therefore flowing red) leaves the heart via tubes known as arteries. Blood returns to the heart (de-oxygenated and faintly blue as seen in the hands and temples) via tubes known as veins.

The chief function of the circulating blood is to supply oxygen and nutritive elements to the billions of tiny cells that make up all body structures, and to remove waste matter from these same cells.

In other words, blood has a two-fold job to perform it is both a food shop and a sewage line for the body. Yet how does this blood that flows away from and back to the heart, tightly contained in "pipes" known as arteries and veins, come into contact with these billions of tiny tissue cells that hunger and thirst incessantly for the oxygen and the food elements that the blood is to bring them?

Nature, as always, has provided a practical way for the cells to receive the vitally needed supplies of oxygen and food from the constantly flowing bloodstream. That way is via capillaries.

Capillaries might be described as tiny, hair-like branches of the main arteries, just as a small twig on a sturdy oak is a ramification of the larger branches and of the huge tree trunk itself. They are fifty times finer than the finest human hair.

The average diameter of a capillary is about 1/3,000 inch, so that the blood can pass through it only one corpuscle at a time, in single file. Remember this fact, for it is all-important in understanding the menace of sludged blood.

So minute is a capillary that it would take 700 of them to make the shaft of a common pin. Each capillary is only about 1/50 of an inch long. Yet, if all the capillaries in the human body were placed end to end, they would form a microscopic tube measuring 35,000 miles.

It is through these almost unbelievably small and innumerable capillaries that normal blood must flow swiftly, one corpuscle at a time, taking about one second to travel the length (1/50 of an inch) of a single capillary.

During this second when the blood is flowing one corpuscle at a time through the tiny capillary, it is performing the mission on which it set out from the heart the mission of bringing food and oxygen to the cells, then gathering up the carbon dioxide and other waste material, leaving the cells both nourished and cleansed.

However, to perform this life-giving mission, the blood does not need to leave the blood vessel. Nature saw to it that the walls of a capillary are extremely thin, consisting of but a single layer of cells, so that oxygen and other nutritive substances from the blood are enabled to filter through this thin wall into the body tissues, while carbon dioxide and other waste products likewise penetrate the capillary wall to enter the bloodstream on their journey back to the lungs and heart via the veins.

After the blood has completed its mission it enters the veins for the return trip to the heart by means of a capillary that generally forms a connecting loop between the other capillaries and the nearby veins.

For a simplified picture of the blood circulation and its mission, let's draw a parallel between feeding the body cells and feeding the inhabitants of a large city.

Food is brought to the city via large trucks and trains (arteries), and then transferred to smaller trucks, wagons and carts (capillaries) for distribution throughout the city, until at last it reaches the home (cell) where it undergoes transformation into usable material and waste products. The waste matter, then, is conveyed away from the home via sewage lines and garbage disposal systems (veins).

Chapter 19

Sick Red Blood Cells

Imagine the chaos and suffering that would descend upon a city if, because of some sudden disaster, the food supply lines and waste disposal systems were prevented from functioning! We have evidence of this, for instance, when a major catastrophe strikes a city without warning, such as happens all too frequently in the flood areas of China or in the earthquake zones of South America.

Let's visualize what would happen and what did happen in bygone days if there were no Red Cross to hasten to the rescue of the stricken city. Not all persons would be affected equally at first; some might have a store of food and fresh water, at least enough to last for several days;

92

while others might be subjected to extreme hunger and thirst almost immediately after the calamity.

Waste and fetid matter would begin accumulating in the streets, causing all manner of horrible diseases and infections.

Those persons suffering most acutely from hunger and thirst would be most readily susceptible to these diseases, and would be those to succumb first. Gradually, the entire populace would begin to feel the pinch of starvation and thirst; one by one they would weaken, and then sicken; one by one they would die off.

The city alone would finally remain a heap of deserted rubble. And thus an entire city would die because, one by one, its inhabitants perished! That is exactly how death comes to the human body. One by one the cells starve, waste away and perish, until gradually the entire body structure of tissues, muscles and bones is destroyed, and life is extinguished!

But why should the cells starve in a body that is fed regularly through its stomach? The people in the stricken city died because they were cut off from food; but why should a cell die for lack of nourishment in a body that receives food at regular intervals?

Even though food is taken into the body via the mouth, there is no assurance that this nourishment will ultimately reach the cell, because sludged blood may have so bogged down the "supply line" that whole masses of cells are starving, literally, in the midst of plenty!

The speed with which the blood "supply line" functions is of paramount importance to the health of the body cells. For example, the blood should make the round trip from the heart to the brain in eight seconds.

A round trip to the legs and toes (the longest route taken by the blood in the circulatory system) should take but a mere 18 seconds. If you don't consider this fast, take out your watch and count off the seconds it takes the blood to make these trips, keeping in mind the complicated route it must travel.

And, in the course of one day, a single red blood cell the largest amount of blood able to pass through the infinitesimally small capillaries at one time should make about 3,000 round trips from heart to lung for oxygen, back to the heart for distribution throughout the tissue cells via the arteries and capillaries, then back again to the heart via the veins.

Imagine the speed and infallibility with which that single red blood cell (along with its trillions of brothers, for there are an estimated 35 trillion red blood cells in the human bloodstream) must travel to make that long, complicated journey 3,000 times a day throughout the maze of arteries, capillaries and veins!

Up until now we have assumed that the blood was healthy and of a normal consistency not sludged and that it was flowing at its normal rate. Yet we know now that blood does not always retain its easy-flowing consistency, that it becomes thick and sludged. How, and why, does this sludge form in the human bloodstream?

When the blood is normal and healthy, the red blood cells float separately in the blood fluid (plasma) like microscopic fish in a rapidly flowing stream. So rapidly do the individual cells move along that they cannot be distinguished even under a powerful microscope.

Freely and independently each tiny red blood cell goes about its mission of transporting oxygen and food substances to the body cells and removing their waste materials.

In fact, a healthy red blood cell is a snob it keeps strictly to itself, never combining with or clinging to any other red blood cell.

But a sick red blood cell or one that has been shocked tends to develop a sticky coating of stagnant mucus that causes it to adhere to other red blood cells, thereby forming clumps of blood. When this occurs, the blood is sludged. His coating of mucus that forms on the ordinarily free-moving red blood cells is entirely foreign to healthy blood.

Chapter 20

Malaria

A disease of long standing malaria, for example causes the red blood cells to develop this mucous film; or it may be a mild disease such as the common cold; or it may even be a wound caused either by an injury or by the surgeon's knife. So far, medical research has discovered over fifty abnormal conditions of the body all the way from the sniffles, hysteria and alcoholism up to severe injury that cause the red blood cells to develop this mucous substance, resulting in clumps of blood in blood vessels designed to hold only liquid, free-flowing life fluid. A red blood cell that develops this sticky coating and clings with other similarly coated cells in sluggish masses is a sickle.

Remember how I have been emphasizing that the blood must flow through the unbelievably tiny capillaries, one cell at a time? This is the reason I have been stressing this point:

If a capillary feeding the tissues of the stomach, let us say, is so tiny it can barely allow the red blood cells to squeeze through one cell at a time, what must happen when a whole clump of red blood cells presents itself at the entrance to a capillary designed by nature to allow passage of the cells in single file only!

What happens to the water supply of a great city (as happened in Chicago several winters ago) when the comparatively small intake pipes in its lakes or reservoirs are suddenly clogged by great masses of ice?

In the case of the city, the water supply is shut off for hours until the ice mass can be blasted and broken up sufficiently to allow water to flow into the pipes. Meanwhile, the city is without water, and consequently suffers a certain degree of hardship.

A poorly functioning organ of the body stomach, intestines, heart, brain, and eyes is a sure indication that not all that organ's tissues are being fed and cleansed of waste materials as efficiently as is necessary to good health.

In other words, sludged blood piles up at the capillary entrances, unable to pass in clumps through the tiny channels, thereby preventing the swift, free flow of life-giving red blood cells in single file.

Gradually sometimes in a matter of hours, sometimes years the tissues die; and when the important tissues, such as those in the heart or brain, are finally killed off because of starvation and decay, the entire body dies!

Chapter 21

Mental Disorders

Much of the blame for mental disorders, as well as cloudy thinking and jittery nerves, can be laid directly at the door of sludged blood. The central nervous system of a psychotic (mentally ill) patient was found to be covered with permanent plugs of clumped red blood cells, so many, in fact, that many of the nerve and brain cells had died from starvation and stagnation, thereby causing the mental disorder.

For this reason, I have been forced to the conclusion that a major percentage of our psychosomatic patients are actually the victims of inadequate nutrition (as we have seen in the previous chapter) complicated further by sludged blood.

A brain and nervous system that does not get the right food, or which cannot be fed because clumps of blood block the capillaries leading to the tissue cells, is bound to react by becoming a brain that cannot think straight or control its emotions, and a nervous system that allows bodily functions to break down!

Premature aging and senility are also suspected of being brought on by dying tissue cells that cannot remain healthy for the sole reason that the blood has become sludged.

Every disease or injury, however, does not form the same amount of sludge in the blood. Nor is the density of the sludge always the same. For instance, in a patient suffering from shock brought on by a wound or injury, the sludge masses become large enough and solid enough to bring about death within five to fifteen hours.

However, in tuberculosis the amount of sludge deposited in the blood is small at first, gradually building up within the arteries over a period of months or years until the clumped blood cells become heavy enough finally to block off entrance to all the vital capillaries.

So-called "secondary anemia" is now recognized as being a direct result of sludged blood. (Secondary anemia is not to be confused with the type of anemia which results from an insufficient number of red blood cells and which respond to treatment by such dietary supplements as iron and chlorophyll.)

Chapter 22

Secondary Anemia

Secondary anemia is always traceable to a direct cause such as hemorrhaging, cancer, weakening discharges or poisoning. Naturally, such serious conditions as these would cause the red blood cells to weaken, form a mucous coating, then to clump together in masses of sludge, thereby shutting off nutriment from whole colonies of vital tissue cells.

Sludged blood presents yet another danger, in addition to causing tissue starvation by blocking the entrances to tiny capillaries. Blood sludge that is allowed to settle in the blood vessels becomes tightly packed, forming large plugs. If and when one of these large plugs of sludged blood is jarred loose and begins moving onward through the bloodstream, it may cause instant death by plugging one of the main arteries. Possibly this is what happens in a great majority of so-called "heart failures."

Certain physicians, as a result of the vital discovery that the health of the body is mirrored in its blood, have begun observing through a special microscope the blood vessels in the eyes of their patients.

This promises to become a valid method of diagnosis, because blood in the eyes comes straight from the heart and flows in a readily accessible part of the body where no surgery is necessary to lay open the arteries.

However, this method of diagnosis is still far from common and, unfortunately, may remain comparatively rare for some time yet. Therefore, it will not be within immediate reach of the average doctor or the average patient.

Why, then, do I consider the discovery of sludged blood as one of the most outstanding advances in modern medicine? Of what value is such knowledge, if it cannot immediately be applied to and practiced by every individual sufferer?

There is hope for these persons in another direction. For some years we have known of an herb that will dissolve stagnant mucus in the human body. We have known that this herb attacks clumps of stagnating mucus in the respiratory tract, in the stomach, intestines and kidneys, dissolving the mucus and allowing it to pass from the body.

We know for certain that this herb is not only an efficient mucus-solvent, but also that it contain beneficial healing substances, such as choline, that enrich the bloodstream, about which we shall learn more in a later chapter. This herb is known as the seeds of fenugreek. Although grown principally in India and the Mediterranean countries, fenugreek seeds are available to every person in this country.

Therefore, it appears that common health sense would indicate the use of this harmless, benevolent herb by any person who has good reason to believe that a certain disease or certain bodily conditions may have caused a mucous coating to form on the red blood cells, thereby slowing down blood circulation to the point where blocks of tissue cells are starving for want of oxygen and nutritive elements.

Any person who is not strictly up to par either mentally or physically may be sure that this is exactly what is happening: sludged blood has so clogged his bloodstream that certain muscles or certain organs become more and more deficient every day, until finally they deteriorate to the point of serious disease.

However, I do not mean to imply that the herb fenugreek is a "miracle" remedy such as is claimed for the sulfa drugs and for penicillin. What I am trying to say is that we know fenugreek seeds have the happy property of being able to dissolve stagnant mucus; further, we know that the coating on the red blood cells which causes them to clump and become sludged is a mucous substance.

Therefore, in the interest of better mental and physical health for everyone, why not give a safe, economical, easily obtainable remedy like this herb a chance at breaking down sludged blood? At least, until the medical laboratories can provide an equally safe and economical remedy for the human body!

Rossie C Pattison

www.ingramcontent.com/pod-product-compliance
Lightning Source LLC
Chambersburg PA
CBHW060421290526
45791CB00002B/846